FROM BUMP TO BABY

GUIDE TO PREGNANCY AND CHILDBIRTH

Camila Mckee

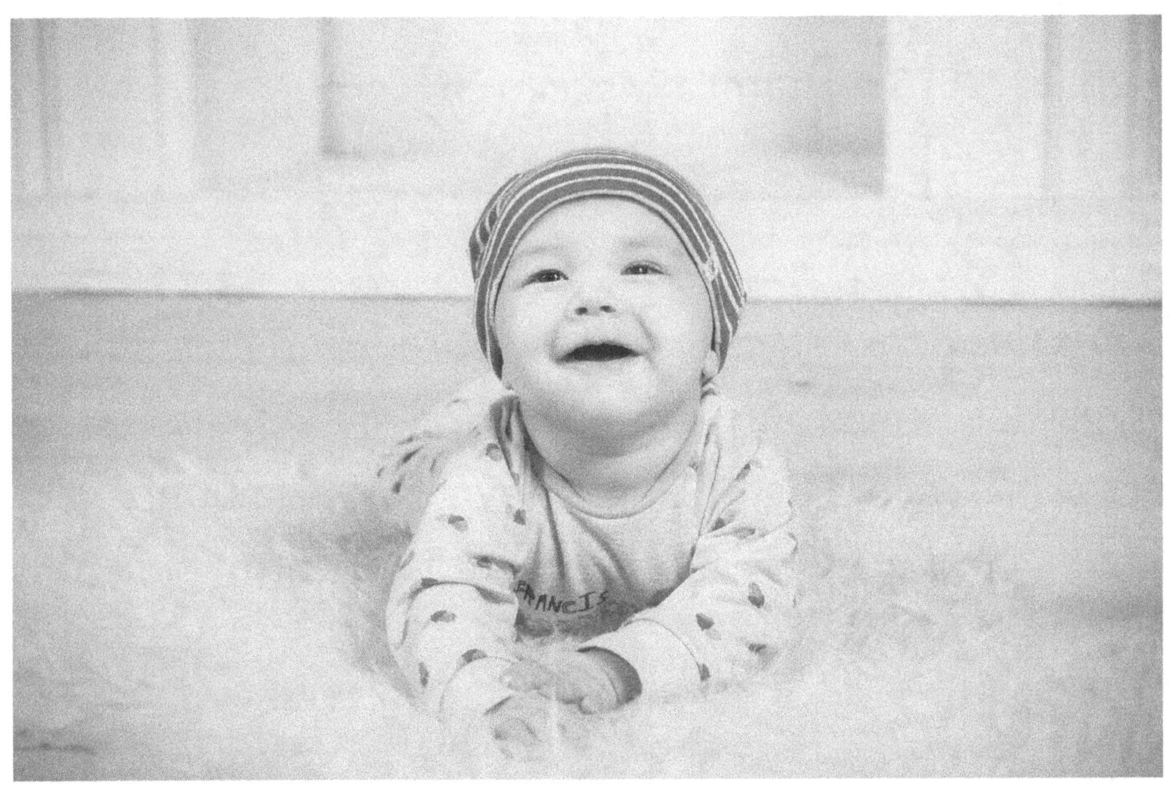

Contents

INTRODUCTION

Welcome to "From Bump to Baby: A Guide to Pregnancy and Childbirth." Congratulations on commencing on this fantastic adventure of bringing new life into the world! Whether you are a first-time parent or have already experienced the pleasures of pregnancy, this book is intended to be your trusted companion, providing important knowledge, advice, and support from the minute you learn you are pregnant until you hold your darling bundle of joy in your arms.

Pregnancy is a spectacular and life-changing experience for a woman. It is a moment of excitement, wonder, and, at times, a fair bit of uncertainty. As a nurse and professional health worker, I understand the plethora of questions and concerns that may emerge throughout this trip. With this book, I want to give you with a thorough resource that will educate you, calm your fears, and help you confidently traverse each stage of pregnancy and labor.

We will dig into every area of pregnancy in "From Bump to Baby," providing practical guidance, evidence-based information, and professional recommendations to help you and your developing baby. We will examine the physical and emotional changes that occur, address common discomforts, and highlight the necessity of a healthy lifestyle and prenatal care from the early stages of conception through the last stages of labor and delivery.

We will also examine the four trimesters of pregnancy, analyzing the growth of your baby as well as the changes occurring inside your own body. Understanding the extraordinary changes that occur at each stage will not only strengthen your bond with your kid, but will also provide you with the knowledge you need to make informed choices about your health and well-being.

Childbirth, without a doubt one of the most profound experiences a woman will ever have, can be both exciting and overwhelming. In this book, we will look at several birthing alternatives and go through the essentials of labor, delivery, and postpartum care. We will discuss pain management approaches, birthing information, and strategies for a successful transition into motherhood.

"From Bump to Baby" will also include advice on how to prepare your house for your newborn, breastfeeding skills and obstacles, the necessity of postpartum care for both mother and baby, and the emotional changes that come with being a parent.

Throughout this book, we will discuss the physical, emotional, and psychological elements of pregnancy, with the goal of fostering a holistic approach to your and your growing family's well-being. It is my earnest goal that the knowledge included within these pages will enable you to make educated choices, appreciate the pleasures, and manage the obstacles that this incredible journey will bring.

Remember that each pregnancy is different, and although this book has a lot of information, it is important to speak with your healthcare practitioner for customized guidance and treatment. Throughout this incredible journey, your healthcare team will be your major source of support and assistance.

So come along with me as we begin on this fantastic journey from bump to baby. Allow this book to be your reliable friend, source of comfort, and guidance to a joyful, healthy, and memorable pregnancy and birthing experience.

CHAPTER 1

Conception and the First Trimester: The Miracle of Life

In this chapter, we will look at the miracle process of conception as well as the amazing changes that occur throughout the first trimester of pregnancy. So, let's get started on this incredible voyage!

1.1 Conception: The Start of Life

Conception is the beginning of new life. It happens when a sperm fertilizes an egg, which results in the development of a single cell known as a zygote. This small zygote has all of the genetic information that will determine your baby's unique qualities, such as eye color, hair texture, and even personality traits. The zygote will divide rapidly, generating an embryo that will embed itself into the uterine lining and grow and develop during the next several months.

1.2 The First Trimester: A Time of Rapid Growth

The first trimester, which lasts from week one to week twelve, is a pivotal and transforming time for both the mother and the developing baby. The embryo quickly grows during this phase, laying the groundwork for all of the key organs, systems, and structures.

1.3 Physical and Emotional Alterations

Expectant moms will go through a variety of physical and mental changes as the embryo implants and develops. Hormonal changes may cause early pregnancy symptoms such as missed periods, breast pain, and morning sickness. During this period, fatigue, frequent urination, and mood changes are also prevalent. It is important to listen to your body and give yourself with the necessary care and rest.

Prenatal Care and a Fit Lifestyle

During the first trimester, early prenatal care is critical. Regular visits to your healthcare professional will safeguard your and your baby's health and well-being. Your healthcare professional will keep track of your development, do required tests and screenings, and advise you on healthy diet, prenatal vitamins, exercise, and avoiding dangerous drugs like as alcohol, smoke, and certain medicines.

1.5 Managing Common Discomforts

Some expecting moms may experience morning sickness, breast changes, food cravings or aversions, and increased urination during the first trimester. While these discomforts might be unpleasant, know that they are usually transient and tend to improve as your pregnancy progresses. We will cover tactics and treatments in this chapter to assist lessen these sensations and make you more comfortable.

1.6 Emotional Health

Pregnancy may cause a broad variety of feelings, including excitement and pleasure as well as fear and mood changes. During this transitional period, it is critical to emphasize your emotional well-being. We will discuss stress management techniques, how to care for your mental health, and how to seek help from your spouse, loved ones, and healthcare professional.

Remember that every pregnancy is different, and each woman's experience may change as you proceed through the first trimester. It is important to have open lines of communication with your healthcare practitioner, to ask questions, and to address any concerns that may develop. You are establishing the groundwork for a healthy and enjoyable pregnancy by taking care of yourself and your developing baby.

In Chapter 2, we'll go further into the second trimester, looking at your baby's growth and development as well as critical concerns for your changing body. So, stay tuned for additional information and thoughts on this great journey from pregnancy to baby!

CHAPTER 2

The Second Trimester: The Blossoming Bump

Let's take a look at the second trimester of pregnancy, sometimes known as the "honeymoon phase" because of the numerous pleasant changes and milestones that occur. So, let us investigate the developing bump and the extraordinary events that occurred throughout this time!

2.1 The Second Trimester: A Time for Growth and Exploration

For expecting moms, the second trimester, which lasts from weeks 13 to 27, is a transforming and thrilling period. The early obstacles of the first trimester generally fade by this point, and the physical and emotional changes become more prominent. During this time, your kid will experience substantial growth and development, and you may find yourself with renewed energy and a stronger bond with your child.

2.2 Baby Development: A Wonderful Journey

Your baby grows and develops rapidly as you proceed through the second trimester. Your baby's organs and systems continue to grow, and his or her characteristics become more distinct. Fingers and toes appear, facial emotions appear, and the skeleton strengthens. Your baby's movements, known as quickening, become more obvious, filling you with delight and anticipation.

2.3 Physical Changes

As your baby grows, your body undergoes visible changes in the second trimester. You may see a distinct baby bump, and your breasts may continue to grow. Morning sickness, increased appetite, and the appearance of a pregnant glow are all frequent physical changes at this period. However, you may face additional difficulties, such as back discomfort, round ligament pain, or stretch marks. We will go through these changes in depth and provide advice on how to deal with any pain.

2.4 Nutritional Requirements and Weight Gain

It is critical to concentrate on fulfilling your dietary requirements and maintaining appropriate weight growth while your baby develops. A healthy diet rich in key nutrients, vitamins, and minerals is critical to your baby's growth and general health. In this chapter, we will address crucial nutritional factors, such as foods to consume and those to avoid, to help you make educated pregnancy decisions.

2.5 Your Baby's Bonding

The second trimester is an excellent time to strengthen your relationship with your developing kid. Feeling their motions and kicks, chatting or singing to them, and even playing music may help them feel connected. We will look at several bonding techniques, such as prenatal courses, meditation, and visualization exercises, to assist enhance the link between you and your child.

2.6 Parenting Preparation

It is normal to begin planning for your baby's birth as the second trimester develops. Making choices regarding birth plans, choosing a healthcare practitioner, and providing a supportive and secure environment for your child are all part of this. We will provide advice on these critical issues, such as delivery alternatives, birthing education, and the need of forming a supporting network of family and friends.

2.7 Emotional Well-Being and Self-Care

Self-care and mental well-being are still important throughout the second trimester. It is critical to emphasize self-care activities that promote relaxation, stress reduction, and mental well-being when your body and emotions experience tremendous changes. We will look at several self-care practices, like as mindfulness exercises, gentle exercises and stretches, and finding moments of calm in the middle of pregnancy's chaos.

We'll get into the third trimester, the last period of pregnancy, in Chapter 3. We will go over the baby's development and positioning, as well as labor and delivery preparations.

CHAPTER 3

The Third Trimester: The Final Countdown

After looking at the first and second trimesters, let's move on to the third trimester of pregnancy. As you approach this stage, you are getting closer to the arrival of your little one. Let's take a look at the major changes and preparations that await you during this changing time.

3.1 The Third Trimester: A Time of Expectation and Planning

The third trimester, which lasts from week 28 until your baby's delivery, is a period of tremendous expectation and preparation. While you manage the physical and emotional changes associated with the final trimester of pregnancy, your baby grows significantly and prepares for life outside the womb.

3.2 Baby's Development and Positioning

During the third trimester, your baby grows rapidly, gaining weight and forming a layer of fat to assist regulate body temperature. As your baby's room in the womb grows more restricted, you may detect more noticeable movements. Your baby's development and position will be monitored by your healthcare professional to ensure their optimum health and preparedness for delivery.

3.3 Labor and Delivery Preparation

As your due date approaches, it is critical to plan for labor and delivery. In this chapter, we will look at several areas of preparation, such as birthing education, making a birth plan, and recognizing the symptoms of labor. We will also go through pain treatment choices such as relaxation methods, breathing exercises, and the use of medication therapies, allowing you to make educated selections based on your preferences and requirements.

3.4 Physical Modifications and Discomforts

Your body endures significant physical changes throughout the third trimester as it prepares for labor and delivery. Increased weariness, backaches, shortness of breath, and swollen ankles and feet are all possible symptoms. We will talk about ways to deal with these discomforts, such as adopting excellent posture, doing light workouts, and wearing maternity apparel and accessories.

3.5 Prenatal Monitoring and Care

During the third trimester, regular prenatal care and monitoring become increasingly more important. Various tests, ultrasounds, and measures will be performed by your healthcare practitioner to monitor your health and the health of your baby. We will discuss the relevance of various tests, such as non-stress testing, Group B strep screening, and fetal movement tracking, to ensure that you have a thorough grasp of the treatment you will get in the last weeks of pregnancy.

3.6 Preparing for Baby's Arrival and Nesting

The third trimester is often associated with a nesting instinct—a desire to provide a secure and caring environment for your kid. We'll go through practical things like setting up the nursery, arranging baby needs, and preparing your hospital bag. This chapter will also go over issues including choosing a doctor, installing a car seat, and becoming acquainted with postpartum care and recovery.

3.7 Accepting Your Emotional Journey

As you near the conclusion of your pregnancy, you may experience a variety of feelings, including excitement, worry, and a great sense of love. We will discuss the emotional components of the third trimester and provide advice on how to deal with anxiety, practice self-care, and seek help from your spouse, loved ones, and healthcare provider. Understanding and accepting the emotional experience can help you approach delivery and parenting with better resilience and confidence.

As you enter the latter stages of your pregnancy, keep in mind that each experience is unique. This chapter will provide you with important information and resources, but you should always consult with your healthcare practitioner for customized advice and treatment.

We shall look at the remarkable process of labor and delivery in Chapter 4. From the first indications of labor through the various phases of labor.

CHAPTER 4

A Birth Experience: Labor, Delivery, and Beyond

In this chapter, we'll go on an incredible adventure through labor, delivery, and the priceless moments that follow. Prepare to obtain a better grasp of the phases of labor and the resources available to you throughout this life-changing event.

4.1 The Birth Miracle: Understanding Labor

Labor refers to the process through which your body prepares for and delivers your baby. It is a remarkable and one-of-a-kind trip that may be both difficult and uplifting. We will look at the three phases of labor in this chapter: early labor, active labor, and the transition period. We will go through the indications of labor, including as contractions and membrane rupture, as well as the necessity of timing contractions to decide when it's time to go to the birthing center or hospital.

4.2 Labor Coping: Pain Management and Comfort Measures

Labor discomfort is an anticipated and normal aspect of the delivery process. This chapter will walk you through several pain management strategies and comfort measures that will assist you in dealing with the severity of contractions. We will investigate a variety of choices to enhance your comfort and well-being throughout labor, including relaxation methods and breathing exercises, massage, hydrotherapy, and the use of birthing tools.

4.3 Labor and Partner Assistance

The presence of a supportive spouse or loved one throughout labor and delivery may make a major impact. We will talk about the role of partners in the delivery process, offering practical advice and ways to assist them provide physical and emotional support. We will also discuss the advantages of hiring a doula or other professional labor support worker to help you have a better delivery experience and advocate for your needs.

4.4 The Birth Experience: Delivery and Immediate Postpartum

The birth of your child is an amazing and life-changing experience. This chapter will look at the various techniques of delivery, such as vaginal birth and cesarean section, and provide information on the procedures, dangers, and advantages of each. We will address the first moments with your infant, skin-to-skin contact, and the basic medical examinations conducted on your baby during the early postpartum period.

4.5 Breastfeeding and Bonding

The bonding process between you and your kid continues after delivery. We will discuss the significance of skin-to-skin contact, early nursing, and the advantages of starting breastfeeding within the first hour after birth. This chapter will go through nursing practices, how to deal with common problems, and how to get help from lactation consultants or breastfeeding support groups.

4.6 Postpartum Recovery and Care

Self-care and support become more important as you enter the postpartum phase. This chapter will discuss many elements of postpartum care, including as physical healing, mental well-being, sleep deprivation management, and the need of creating a support network. We will talk about the changes that occur in your body after delivery and provide you advice on how to care for your infant while also taking care of yourself.

4.7 Accepting Your New Parental Role

Becoming a parent is a life-changing event that comes with it a lot of pleasure, love, and responsibility. We will discuss the emotional changes that occur with motherhood, such as the baby blues and postpartum depression, as well as the need of getting assistance and support when required. This chapter will discuss how to strengthen the parent-child link, make time for self-care, and embrace the difficulties and benefits of this new chapter in your life.

Remember that every birth experience is unique as you prepare for the journey of labor, delivery, and afterwards. While this chapter gives a complete overview, it is critical that you speak with your healthcare practitioner and develop a birth plan that aligns with your preferences.

CHAPTER 5

Pregnancy Care: Diet, Exercise, and Coping Strategies

Let us now look at some important parts of nourishing your pregnancy, such as eating a good food, participating in safe workouts, and dealing with the physical and emotional changes that come with this life-changing adventure.

5.1 Nourishing Your Body: A Pregnancy Diet That Works

Proper diet is essential throughout pregnancy to support your baby's growth and development as well as your general health. In this chapter, we'll go over the essential nutrients your body need throughout pregnancy, such as folic acid, iron, calcium, and omega-3 fatty acids. We will look at a balanced diet that includes fruits, vegetables, whole grains, lean meats, and healthy fats. We will also discuss typical pregnant desires and aversions, as well as techniques for selecting smart eating choices while enjoying in moderation.

5.2 Maintaining a Healthy Weight Gain Balance

Weight gain is a normal and necessary component of pregnancy, but it is critical to maintain a healthy balance. We will look at criteria for safe weight increase during pregnancy depending on your pre-pregnancy BMI. While some weight gain is normal, excessive weight gain may raise the risk of problems, and insufficient weight gain may have an influence on your baby's development. We will provide advice on how to manage weight gain via a mix of healthful food and moderate activity.

5.3 Pregnancy Exercise That Is Safe

Regular physical exercise while pregnant has various advantages for both you and your baby. We will examine safe exercise alternatives in this chapter, like as walking, swimming, prenatal yoga, and low-impact aerobics. We'll also talk about how pelvic floor exercises may help you support your body throughout pregnancy and prepare for birth and delivery. Before beginning or maintaining any fitness regimen during pregnancy, always speak with your healthcare professional to confirm that it is safe for both you and your baby.

5.4 Adjusting to Physical Changes: Body Image and Comfort

Pregnancy causes major bodily changes, and each woman's experience is different. We'll talk about typical body image issues and give coping skills to help you appreciate and enjoy the changes your body is going through. We will discuss techniques to assist your physical and mental comfort throughout pregnancy, from managing stretch marks and varicose veins to selecting comfortable clothes and footwear.

5.5 Tips and Remedies for Managing Pregnancy Discomforts

During pregnancy, you may experience a variety of discomforts such as heartburn, back pain, and swollen ankles. We will explore practical methods and natural therapies to ease these discomforts in this chapter, including as appropriate body posture, warm baths, and the usage of pregnant pillows. However, before taking any treatments or drugs during pregnancy, please with your healthcare professional to confirm they are safe for you and your baby.

5.6 Emotional Health: Managing Pregnancy Hormones

Pregnancy hormones may have an effect on your emotions and mental health. This chapter will look at coping techniques for dealing with mood swings, anxiety, and stress throughout pregnancy. We'll talk about the value of self-care, such as relaxation methods, mindfulness practices, and getting emotional assistance from loved ones or professional counselors.

5.7 Preparing for Your Baby's Arrival: Nesting and Beyond

The anticipation of your baby's coming may become stronger as your pregnancy continues. We'll talk about nesting and the natural desire to prepare your house for your new baby. This chapter will walk you through practical preparations including setting up the nursery, gathering baby necessities, and making a birth plan. We'll also talk about the importance of postpartum preparation and creating a support network in the weeks and months after delivery.

Remember that caring for your pregnancy includes your physical, emotional, and mental well-being.

CHAPTER 6

Pregnancy, Birth, and Beyond: A Safe and Healthy Environment

In this chapter, we'll talk about how important it is to create a safe and healthy environment for yourself and your kid throughout pregnancy, delivery, and the transition to parenting. Let's have a look at the major issues and practical ideas for boosting well-being throughout this transitional period.

6.1 Creating a Nurturing Environment: A Safe Home

The cornerstone of your family's well-being is your house. It is important to provide a safe and caring environment for yourself and your kid throughout pregnancy and afterwards. This chapter will go over many areas of home safety, such as babyproofing, establishing a calm sleeping environment, and keeping your house clean and toxin-free. We will go through possible risks to be aware of and practical ideas for keeping your house safe and pleasant.

6.2 Putting Together a Birth Support Team: Selecting a Healthcare Provider

It is critical to choose a healthcare practitioner that shares your birth wishes and offers thorough prenatal care. We will cover many sorts of healthcare professionals, such as obstetricians, midwives, and doulas, as well as the advantages and disadvantages of each. We'll also talk about the value of open communication, trust, and shared decision-making with your healthcare team.

6.3 Birth Preferences: Investigating Your Options

The location of your birth might have a significant impact on your birth experience. This chapter will look at various birth environments, such as hospitals, birthing centers, and home births. We will go through the benefits and drawbacks of each choice, allowing you to make an educated decision based on your tastes and medical requirements.

6.4 Making a Birth Plan: Communicating Your Expectations

A birth plan is a written document that specifies your labor, delivery, and postpartum care choices. This chapter will walk you through the process of developing a birth plan, including topics such as pain management preferences, interventions, breastfeeding objectives, and infant care options. As you navigate the delivery experience, we will highlight the value of flexibility and open communication with your healthcare team.

6.5 The Role of Birth Companions and Doulas

A supportive birth partner or doula may greatly improve your delivery experience. We will discuss birth partners' and doulas' roles and duties, including emotional support, physical comfort measures, and advocacy. This chapter will help you and your birth support team communicate and collaborate effectively with your healthcare provider.

6.6 Infant CPR and First Aid: Keeping Your Child Safe

Knowing basic infant CPR (Cardiopulmonary Resuscitation) and first aid procedures is critical for safeguarding your baby's safety and well-being. This chapter will provide you an introduction of baby CPR and first aid standards, such as how to deal with choking, breathing crises, and common injuries. We'll also talk about how important it is to take a certified baby CPR and first aid course to obtain practical skills and confidence.

6.7 Parenting Preparation: Education and Support

Gaining information and finding assistance as you prepare to become a parent is crucial. This chapter will discuss the significance of parental education, which includes birthing courses, breastfeeding classes, and infant care seminars. We'll go through the advantages of joining parental support groups, obtaining advice from experienced parents, and gaining access to trustworthy resources to assist you navigate the pleasures and difficulties of motherhood.

You are taking proactive actions to ensure the well-being of yourself and your baby by providing a safe and healthy environment, assembling a supportive birth team, and obtaining necessary information and skills. In Chapter 7, we will look at the postpartum period, sometimes known as the fourth trimester.

The Postpartum Period in the Fourth Trimester

We shall now look at the fourth trimester—the time after delivery. We will discuss the physical recuperation, emotional changes, and practical elements of caring for yourself and your infant during this transforming period as you start on your journey as a new parent.

7.1 An Overview of the Fourth Trimester

The fourth trimester is the period after delivery during which both you and your baby adapt to your new responsibilities. This chapter will offer an overview of the fourth trimester's distinctive qualities, such as physical recovery following delivery, emotional adaptations of early parenting, and your newborn's quick growth and requirements.

7.2 Physical Recovery: Self-Care and Healing

Your body goes through a wonderful healing and recovery process after delivery. This chapter will go over typical bodily changes such as postpartum hemorrhage, perineal pain, and breast engorgement. During this time of transition, we will look at ways to promote healing, manage pain, and prioritize self-care.

7.3 Breastfeeding: Creating a Nurturing Bond

Breastfeeding has various advantages for both you and your child. This chapter will walk you through the fundamentals of breastfeeding, including as posture and latching practices, milk supply establishment, and detecting hunger and satiety signals. We will explore typical difficulties and provide advice on how to get help from lactation consultants and nursing support organizations.

7.4 Newborn Care: Providing for Your Baby's Needs

Caring for a baby can be both exciting and exhausting. This chapter will go through the fundamentals of infant care, such as washing, diapering, calming methods, and safe sleeping habits. We'll talk about understanding your baby's signs, encouraging bonding and attachment, and creating a caring routine that promotes your baby's growth and well-being.

7.5 Postpartum Emotional Well-Being: A Postpartum Rollercoaster

The postpartum period is associated with a wide variety of feelings, which are sometimes referred to as "baby blues" or postpartum mental disorders. This chapter will look at the emotional changes you may go through, how to recognize indicators of postpartum depression and anxiety, and techniques for self-care and getting help. We will stress the significance of addressing your mental health while caring for your infant.

7.6 Relationship Nurturing: Partner, Family, and Support

Your whole family will be adjusting throughout the postpartum period. During this transitional period, this chapter will explore ways for fostering connections with your spouse, siblings, and extended family members. We'll talk about how important it is to communicate openly, share responsibilities, and seek help from loved ones and support networks.

7.7 Self-Care and Well-Being: Putting Your Needs First

Self-care is essential throughout the postpartum time. This chapter will emphasize the significance of self-care, which includes proper rest, diet, and exercise. We'll go through practical ways for dealing with sleep loss, making time for self-care, and getting help to preserve your physical, emotional, and mental well-being as a new parent.

Remember that each parent and baby's experience is unique as you traverse the fourth trimester. This chapter offers you with important information and resources, but it is critical that you talk with your healthcare physician and seek specific assistance and support from trusted specialists.

We will reflect on your journey from pregnancy to motherhood in the last chapter and give closing remarks and resources to help you as you embrace this great chapter of your life.

CHAPTER 8

Reflections and Closing Thoughts on Parenthood

As you near the conclusion of your life-changing adventure, it's time to reflect on your experiences, celebrate your victories, and provide some last thoughts and advice as you embrace the magnificent role of parenting.

8.1 Embracing Parenthood: A Love and Growth Journey

Becoming a parent is a profound and life-changing event. It is a journey full of love, joy, hardships, and personal development. In this chapter, we urge you to reflect on your individual path, enjoying the moments of connection, lessons learned, and progress as you transitioned into motherhood.

8.2 Cherishing Memories: Preserving and Capturing Moments

Time flies, and as a parent, you will experience your child's extraordinary growth and development. This chapter encourages you to appreciate and preserve important memories by photographing them, documenting them, and making mementos. Consider how important it is to memorialize your experience and leave a legacy that you and your kid may look back on with pleasure and thankfulness.

8.3 Words of Wisdom: Lessons Learned and Wisdom Shared

It is beneficial to rely on the experiences and knowledge of others as you begin on your parenting journey. We give advise from parents who have travelled a similar route in this chapter. We discuss how to raise a caring and supportive family, achieve balance in the middle of parenthood's obligations, and find pleasure in the mundane. Remember that no parent has all the answers, and it is OK to seek advice and help when necessary.

8.4 Self-Compassion and Development: Accepting Imperfection

Parenthood is a continual process of learning and development, but it's important to realize that no one is perfect. In this chapter, we'll talk about the importance of self-compassion, accepting flaws, and embracing the messiness and unpredictability of parenting. We urge you to celebrate your victories, learn from your setbacks, and create a growth and resilience attitude.

8.5 Relationship Care: Love, Communication, and Connection

It's critical to focus and cultivate your connections with your spouse, family, and friends as you embark on motherhood. This chapter looks at ways to keep the lines of communication open, nurture love and connection, and strike a balance between your responsibilities as parents and people. We stress the significance of self-care and establishing a support network that pulls you up in both happy and sad times.

8.6 Gratitude and Mindfulness: Finding Joy in the Present Parenthood may be a tornado of obligations and emotions, and it's easy to get engrossed in the hustle and bustle of everyday life. We urge you to practice thankfulness and mindfulness as skills for finding pleasure in the present moment in this chapter. We talk about the importance of stopping, enjoying tiny miracles, and relishing the ephemeral phases of your child's development.

8.7 Keeping the Journey Going: Resources and Help

As you finish this handbook, keep in mind that your journey as a parent is far from over. This chapter includes a list of resources, such as books, websites, and support groups, to help you continue your journey of learning and discovery. It emphasizes the necessity of getting help, interacting with other parents, and finding credible information as you manage your child's and family's changing needs.

Finally, we want to congratulate you on your pregnancy journey and thank you for your dedication to creating a supportive and loving environment for your kid. Parenthood is an incredible experience full with unlimited chances for love, development, and connection. May your trip be filled with wonderful memories, deep delight, and happiness.

CONCLUSION

Embracing Parenthood's Miracles

Congratulations! You have completed "From Bump to Baby: A Guide to Pregnancy and Childbirth." We've looked at the amazing phases of pregnancy, the pleasures and trials of delivery, and the transforming transition into motherhood. We provide some closing words and encouragement as you begin on this wonderful chapter of your life as you reflect on all you have learned and experienced.

Parenthood is a remarkable gift—a journey that will put your strength, resilience, and capacity for love to the test in unexpected ways. It's a kaleidoscope of feelings, a careful mix of enormous delight and vulnerable times. It is a trip that will reveal your true nature, where you will learn new levels of compassion, patience, and selflessness.

Remember that you are not alone when you embark on motherhood. Lean on your support network, seek expert advice, and connect with other parents who understand the lovely turmoil that is raising a kid. Parenthood is a communal experience with a lot of information and wisdom to be shared.

Remember to be kind with yourself in the middle of the sleepless nights, difficult times, and tornado of duties. Accept flaws and make place for development and self-compassion. You are going on a lifetime path of learning and discovery, and you will make mistakes. However, each blunder is a chance for both you and your kid to improve.

Find delight in the current moment. The first steps, those little fingers wrapped around yours, the contagious giggles—parenthood is full of ephemeral moments. Accept the beauty of ordinary life, the simplicity of shared laughing, and the awe of seeing your kid discover the world. Be present in these times, appreciate them, and make lasting memories.

Maintain your connections. Parenthood might seem all-consuming at times, but remember to nurture your love and connection with your spouse, family, and friends. Openly communicate with one another, support one another through highs and lows, and create places for laughter, closeness, and shared experiences. You will lay a solid foundation for your child's journey together.

Above all, keep in mind that love is at the core of parenting. Your love for your kid will lead you through the difficulties and brighten the route ahead. Accept the wonders that unfold before your eyes—the first word, the soft touch, and the accomplishments. Keep in mind the blessing of experiencing a new life bloom under your care and direction.

As you finish this guide, we hope it has given you useful knowledge, inspiration, and confidence. But keep in mind that no handbook can entirely prepare you for the complexities of your own trip. Trust your intuition, pay attention to your child's needs, and let the love in your heart to lead you.

May your parenting path be filled with awe, joy, and the highest kinds of love. Accept the marvels that await you because they are the best presents you will ever get.